A FOODIE'S GUIDE *to* JUICE FASTING

JULIANNE DOWSE

BALBOA.
PRESS
A DIVISION OF HAY HOUSE

Balboa Press books may be ordered through booksellers or by contacting:

Balboa Press
A Division of Hay House
1663 Liberty Drive
Bloomington, IN 47403
www.balboapress.com
1 (877) 407-4847

Because of the dynamic nature of the Internet, any web addresses or links contained in this book may have changed since publication and may no longer be valid. The views expressed in this work are solely those of the author and do not necessarily reflect the views of the publisher, and the publisher hereby disclaims any responsibility for them.

The author of this book does not dispense medical advice or prescribe the use of any technique as a form of treatment for physical, emotional, or medical problems without the advice of a physician, either directly or indirectly. The intent of the author is only to offer information of a general nature to help you in your quest for emotional and spiritual well-being. In the event you use any of the information in this book for yourself, which is your constitutional right, the author and the publisher assume no responsibility for your actions.

Print information available on the last page.

ISBN: 978-1-4525-2774-1 (sc)
ISBN: 978-1-4525-2775-8 (e)

Balboa Press rev. date: 03/30/2015

CONTENTS

"The spirit desires to remain with its body, because, without the organic instruments of that body, it can neither act, nor feel anything."
~ Leonardo da Vinci (1452 - 1519)

Leonardo da Vinci was an Italian artist of the Renaissance who was an architect, painter, sculptor, inventor, engineer and writer. He is known for his enduring works "The Last Supper" and "Mona Lisa."

"When it comes to taking care of your health, my wish for you is that you'll simply seek the truth before just blindly handing yourself over to a credentialed expert. Do your homework - and then and only then, choose a path that seems logical, reasonable and right for you."
~ Don Tolman (Born 16 October 1946)

Don Tolman is known as the Whole Food Cowboy and an expert in nutrition and natural medicine. Don has spent well over 40 years investigating cultures that are long-lived and basically disease-free. He has lectured at medical symposiums and travels the world sharing the message of 'do it yourself self-care'.

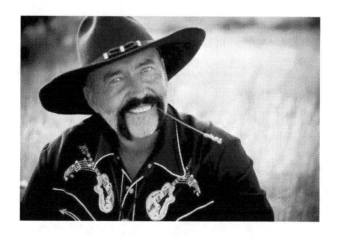

Foreword by Don Tolman

I love the Simplicity and Sacred Healing Knowledge that Julianne (whose name means Young and Pure), presents as a Foodie's Guide to the 'Wonders of Juice' Fasting.

Most if not all who read this synopsis of Ancient Self-Healing Wisdom will realize that the Plant Foods on this Planet are meant to be the only Medicine we as Humans ever eat or drink, because they awaken and strengthen the Powers of the Body to Heal, Recover, Restore and Maintain Energy, Health, Happiness and Pleasure.

The Self-Healing Revolution is here.

We need to realize that Pharmacy is legal distribution of poisons to try and target symptoms, not healing.

Nature's Farmacy comes to us from Father Sun and Mother Earth as Light, gases, liquids and solids.

Ancient cultures of Healing used words like sap, sop, sip, soups, succus, suck and pi (later pie), which eventually formed into the english, Juice.

Osira-peth, a Juice and Diet Healer at the Temple of On in Heliopolis (later called Moses from the waters/liquids), taught fasting on waters and juice for Healing.

Luu, luw, lew, loo, juju, juiu and eventually jews meant to 'Strengthen on the Waters' or jewsus/juices. The blood of juices/jesus was the liquids extracted from grapes (hence wine as a sacred drink or sacrament), tomatoes, watermelons and hundreds more fruits. This was the collective wisdom of the ages for restoration, healing and social pleasures.

Today the fascination with healing through foods and juices is stronger than ever. Pharmaceutical articles have and continue, to this day, to bash this Ancient Knowledge.

Anyone who does juice fasting and shares their results as testimonials is bringing a Noble Art into the House of Modern research Science. More and more doctors and nurses are waking up to the truest truth facts: that drugs and surgeries are not the only path to recovery and health and in fact the Cut, Burn and Poisoning of today's medical world are doing more harm than good.

Here is a quote that might shock you. It is from Sir William Osler - widely called the "Father of Modern Medicine" - who was Head of the Department of Medicine at John Hopkins at the turn of the 19th century. In talking to medical students about the famous quote attributed to Hippocrates "First do no harm", he said "One of the first duties of the physician is to educate the masses not to take medical drugs".

Medical journals have published studies that show if a person eats quarter of an apple a day, they cut their risk of heart disease in half. "An apple a day keeps the doctor away" turns out to be a truest truth. Juice fasting has been proven to clear and heal over 300 different kinds of diseases.

I recommend Julianne's 'Foodie's Guide to Juice Fasting' 100%!!!

Please read and ponder and reflect on what this book brings to you. Then do your own scientific research by actually doing a juice fast or at least adding Julianne's juice recipes into your daily diet.

Thank you again Julianne. You are blessing lives with Life, Liberty and Freedom from disease, as they find and pursue Happiness.

CowBoy Don Tolman the Whole Foodie Medicine Man.

"I thought I was learning to live; I was only learning to die."
    ~ Leonardo da Vinci (1452 - 1519)

Leonardo da Vinci was an Italian artist of the Renaissance who was an architect, painter, sculptor, inventor, engineer and writer. He is known for his enduring works "The Last Supper" and "Mona Lisa."

CHAPTER 1

Introduction

Oh my God, who would have thought, me, a foodie, would be here writing a book on fasting?

This has to be the opposite of what I love most in my life. Okay, so it's my husband, Gary, and our two gorgeous Labradors first, but hey, food is definitely a very close second. I love food. I love cooking it, eating it, researching it, discovering it, and experimenting with it. I love the smell and the experiences you get because of it, and it's pretty much what dictates most of what I do and where I go in life. "Oh, let's go here; it's a food festival," or "Wanna check out the farmers' market?" or my favourite, "Let's go check out this new restaurant—I've heard their desserts are divine!" Yes, yes, yes—a foodie I definitely am.

So what on earth is a person who loves food so much doing writing a book about going without the very thing she claims to love? Well, it's like this: I got tired of the people around me dying.

Grandparents, parents, sister, cousin, aunties; lots of death, lots of sickness, lots of people thinking they were doing the right thing, the safe thing, the good and healthy thing, only to find out they weren't. Not even close. In a nutshell: "They just didn't know what they didn't know."

My story goes like this: Once upon a time, there lived a fairly typical girl in a pretty typical life. She worked in the middle of a big city in a really big office building, and she looked forward to her weekends and life outside "those walls" more than anything. She was a party girl and loved being social and going out dancing and drinking and having fun with her friends. She was young, child-free, living on her own, and having the time of her life!

This typical girl came from a big family, seven children in all, pretty much all raised by a single mum. "Hang on a minute, seven children is hardly typical," I hear you say. Yes, in this day and age it might not be, but where I come from and when I grew up, big families were the norm.

This typical girl, with her very big family, with all of her sisters and brother now married and all with children (so it's extra big now) all basically followed the same path. They all grew up with a family doctor, and regular visits were just part of life—like going to the dentist or getting your hair cut.

Whatever the doctor said went. If the doctor said you needed to get a flu shot, you did. If he said you needed to take a course of antibiotics, you did. If he said you needed to take some tests, you did. And if he said you needed to go home and rest, that advice was followed too.

The doctor played a very important role within the typical girl's family. The years went by with the doctor always listened to and everyone always doing as they were told. The doctor's words were never questioned, never put to the test. They existed to be that truth, the one voice that had only your best interest at heart.

This was all well and good until people close to the girl, people she loved more than anything, started getting sick and actually didn't get better. They might have for a little bit, but soon enough something else would be wrong, and off to the doctor they would go again.

It played out like this: The unsuspecting relatives would go to the doctor with a symptom, one that had been getting progressively worse each month, each year. They would go, already fearful, already knowing they should have done something sooner, something to ward off the inevitable, something to alleviate the downward spiral. So they went to the doctor—almost with tail between legs—saying, "I've got such-and-such, and it's been there for ages, and I haven't paid it much attention" (although they had thought about it constantly for days, weeks, months, and sometimes years).

Then the process would begin. Test after test, analysis after analysis, until a conclusion was determined and a treatment plan would follow.

That's when typical girl would get called in. She, along with the rest of her family, would gather around and support whoever happened to be going through whatever treatment had been decided. They would do what they could do—which wasn't much.

Relative after relative would go down this path—until they stopped getting better. Their symptom became many symptoms, and there weren't enough drugs or things they could do to alleviate the pain or the inevitability of their grave situation.

So, typical girl found herself asking, "What is going on? Why do all the people I cherish most in this world get sick and die? Is this it? Is this how life plays out?" Cancer one in two, diabetes following a very close second, heart conditions—is this it? You work through everything in life—relationship bust-ups, job failures, weight issues, self-esteem issues, depression, bullying, money issues—all of those painful experiences that helped you grow like nothing else, only to get sick and die?

You're kidding right, surely there is more? Surely there is a better way? And so, this is where the real story begins. It's about why I, your typical girl with a fairly typical life, made a decision to find a better way, to seriously find a better way and to break the pattern that was being handed down like a 'prized parcel of land' from generation to generation to generation. Yes, this is where typical girl made a decision that enough was enough.

And, whilst she couldn't change the past, she couldn't bring people back who had died, nor change what everyone else did with, and in, their lives with regards to health and sickness, she absolutely *could* change what she did and how she viewed health and looked after her own body.

Now you have some context as to why I have been unconsciously propelled into this space. I haven't found my way here because of any real sickness; I haven't discovered a lump, I haven't had any tests, nor has a psychic told me I really need to do something about my energy field. I am just a typical girl who enjoys life and all the bounty it offers, and I am not someone whose driving force comes from a diagnosis.

The passion I have comes from the very sad fact that by the time I was thirty-six, I had already witnessed the death of my mother, father, sister, aunty, cousin, and both sets of grandparents. The thing is, every one of them died by their own hand; they all had stuff going on in their bodies that they truly could have prevented through making diet and lifestyle changes. All of these beautiful people who were a part of my life, who had stories to share, lives to live, and families to be part of, died because they were all just too scared and—sad to say—too ignorant.

They blindly followed when their hearts told them otherwise; they ignored their own bodies when little symptoms led to bigger wake-up symptoms—led to death. They didn't understand that their bodies were trying to communicate to them, working to keep them alive with every lump, bump, rash, cough, ache, pain. They didn't understand that their bodies were helping them survive, not trying to kill them. And so they perished, but not in a romantic die-in-your-sleep way; they suffered horribly for months and sadly even years. When their time was done, they didn't even have bodies that could allow an open coffin at their funeral. Only the eyes of those close to them, who loved them regardless of their withered frame, their now-unrecognisable features, and their dark and lifeless eyes, would see them in this state.

Each and every one of these family members just didn't take responsibility for his or her own body; they chose to stay ignorant and let fear run the show.

That may sound harsh, but the stripped-bare truth is that they just didn't know what they didn't know, and in the end, their well-meaning doctors ran out of drugs and options to help them. By the time they had surrendered to trying nature's medicine, it was far too late; death had already taken hold.

In this day and age, we have far more options. We only have to ask better questions, and we will get a myriad of responses. The thing is, when you are scared and tired and in pain, that can be the hardest thing in the world to do—to ask better questions. So you go along with "whatever is best"—but for whom? Is it best for the doctor you are seeing, your partner, your family, or your well-meaning friends?

Often, the decision is too hard and overwhelming to make, so you just do what you do, with the limited knowledge you have, and those close to you support you as best they can.

But what if we really understood what was going on in our own bodies? What if we knew what to do when we noticed the first signs of trouble? What if we trusted that our bodies could actually heal themselves if they were supported on the journey?

So that is the driving force behind this book, the book I never ever thought that I would write. It's my way of reaching out to you, to your friend, to your mother, sister, cousin and aunty; it's my way of inspiring you to walk a different path and to be open to another way. I also write it to challenge and expand your thoughts and get you to stop for a moment, take a breath and connect in.

It's me, your typical girl, wanting SO much more for you and your life and for all of those who are connected with you. Just a typical girl with a typical life who has discovered (or is that remembered?) an ancient truth we all have within us which is to heal and rejuvenate our body. It's me reaching out to you from a place of wisdom to say:

"Hey, what if there was another way, what if this amazing body of ours could actually heal itself, yep, wouldn't that be nice?"

So, welcome to the world of juice fasting by a typical girl.

"There is nothing more ancient than truth"
~ Rene Descartes (1596 – 1650)

A French mathematician, scientist, and philosopher
who promoted the development of a new science
grounded in observation and experiment.

CHAPTER 2

The fast story

What on earth is fasting all about? Is it just some spiritual thing that doesn't have a place in the 'real' world? Surely it can't be good to go without food, you will surely die - won't you?

Okay, here's what I have discovered about fasting. To fast is to make strong!

When I fast-en something to something else, it makes it stronger, it increases the strength of the original thing and so, when we fast we make our body stronger.

That doesn't make sense to most people as most people know that to fast means to go without, to abstain from all of the things you love, how can that make you strong? Well, hang here with me for a bit and I will show you.

There are loads of different fasts you can do, from taking in nothing but air to nothing but watermelon and everything in between, but they all have a few things in common - it's a diet and lifestyle change. It is time out from your standard routine (whatever that is), to give your body an opportunity to do what it is best at: Rid, Repair and Rejuvenate!

Now whilst there are loads and loads of fasts that you can do, this book is about juice fasting - the sweet nectar of fruit and vegetables - or more deliciously named, 'liquid sunlight'. It's all about giving your body juices that are simple and easy on your digestive system, which provide your body with everything it needs to get the job done and perform at its optimal best!

So, why do it?

For most people, fasting of any sort usually kicks in when illness is present. But, truth be told, in ancient times, periods of fasting were built into normal life. There was a lovely balance between work, rest and play. Which means that in our modern super-charged world, where often balance is hard to come by, we need fasting more than ever before.

Why is it so important to include a form of fasting into our life? It's all about good health and longevity - that's why!

Everyone knows that animals stop eating if they get sick. If you have a pet, you will know this to be true. In fact dogs will go out and eat grass to make themselves throw up if they have something in their stomach that isn't good for them - it's innate within them. Babies are the same. They go off their food and tend to sleep a lot more. It's like they are hard-wired to do this even as very young beings. Thing is, they know how to support their body. They know that going without food gives their busiest system - their digestive system - a break, so that all of that energy which usually goes towards breaking down food can be utilised elsewhere in the body to rid, repair and rejuvenate.

The body loves having the opportunity to do some internal cleaning because it truly loves to run at its best, all of the time, not just some of the time. So, when we give it a break from digesting food, we give all of those cells that pretty much run flat chat all day a chance to divert their energy elsewhere and go on a 'cleaning frenzy'.

No matter what type of fast you do, they all do pretty much the same thing, which is cleanse toxins from our body. Once that is well underway, the cells also do some other really cool stuff: they cruise around looking for any sites in need of some repair and then what happens as a result of this is even cooler - you have way more fully functioning cells doing their thing, which means you now have loads more energy to do what you love to do, which is live life! All of this happens quite by magic really, but the actual fact is the micro-nutrients in fresh, cold-pressed juice provide all the energy to stimulate the detoxification process, by clearing waste from your systems. This is an important process as it allows our body to breathe and naturally cleanse itself. As I said, it is innate within us!

Fasting as a way to heal dates back thousands of years. Not only that, many religions, including Christianity, Judaism, and Eastern religions still use fasting as a healing process for spiritual purification and communion with God. Fasting effects not only our physical being, but our mental, emotional, and spiritual self as well.

It's like when you put your car in and they do a total overhaul: tyres are checked, oil and water levels topped up, new wipers are put on etc. Your body is YOUR vehicle, it houses your spirit and every now and then, depending on your lifestyle (how hard you drive it), you just need to give it a service. Juice fasting is an easy and effective way to do that.

I can't imagine our kidneys saying "Hey, I've been working 24/7 for 40 years now. I reckon I am entitled to some long service leave," and off they go into the sunset with the liver in tow!!!

No, none of our organs do that. They plug away 24/7 without a break, mostly not really getting what they need to do their job (kinda like a chef in a kitchen without any modern conveniences, you get the job done, but…how stressful can it be to not have the right tools or products at your disposal).

So, after all of that hard work on a constant basis, with no real break, all of our organs become a bit tired, overused, inflamed and pretty much just need a moment to repair and recharge.

Fasting gives our body a chance to clean up its act because it is not expending energy towards the digestive organs. When we fast, all of the chaos created at a cellular level from a bad diet, exposure to toxins in our environment and an unhealthy lifestyle gets to be released - kinda like having a super huge spring clean, only internally!

Here are some cool trailblazers:

- Pythagoras (ancient Greek philosopher and mathematician) understood the impact that a clean body has on the brain and insisted that all prospective students fast for six weeks before he would tutor them.
- After Gandhi (father of the Indian independence movement) was assassinated at 77, his doctors commented that his organs looked like those of a 35 year old. Their only explanation was the extensive fasting he had done.
- Plutarch (ancient Greek historian) said, "Instead of medicine, fast for a day."

This remains excellent advice. At the first sign of a cold or flu, or any other acute illness, if you will take to your bed and cease eating, your body will have the opportunity to cleanse and heal itself much more quickly.

The benefits that are afforded to us via fasting are numerous and varied, from heightened spiritual awareness and relaxation of the body, mind, and emotions, to a sense of letting go of pain from the past and developing a positive attitude towards the present.

Fasting is not magic, though it often seems so. It is simply nature's way of allowing the organism the best possible conditions in which to cleanse and heal itself.

"Wisdom begins in wonder."
~ Socrates (circa 470 BC – 399 BC)

Socrates was a classical Greek (Athenian) philosopher who is credited as one of the founders of Western philosophy. Socrates' wisdom was limited to an awareness of his own ignorance, he always claimed he 'knew nothing'. Socrates invited others to concentrate on friendships and a sense of true community as the best way for people to grow together as a populace.

CHAPTER 3

Baby steps

One of my philosophies in life is "Make the rules so you win". What this means is, don't bite off more than you can chew; or another way to look at this is, always put yourself in the best possible place for guaranteed victory.

For instance, if you are a meat eater and you have been thinking a vegetarian diet would be much healthier for you, then going cold turkey (pardon the pun) and stopping all meat consumption from day one is probably not going to give you the best results.

Start by first introducing more vegetarian meals into your diet. Replace one meal, then two, then a whole day of meals and see how you feel. It's always much easier to do something when we are not feeling pressured, so just start slowly and build up to it. You may find you enjoy the variety and different flavours you get from eating vegetarian, but you might also find you miss eating meat too much and hey, that's okay - you need to do what is right for you.

Whilst I've been a veggie for years now, it actually took me many years to become that. First Gary and I stopped eating steak, then we only ate organic meat, then we only ate chicken, then it was only fish….now, it's just fruit and veggies, which we love more than anything!

The same goes with juice fasting. Start slowly introducing juices into your diet (unless of course you have got some major health issues going on, then that's a different story).

But, I am hoping you are reading this because you want to incorporate juice fasting in your self-care regime and you want to explore what juice fasting is all about before you undertake it. If so, then great – here are some easy ways to do that.

Start by picking some 'tame' juices, like watermelon and mint or carrot, apple and celery. Don't start off with juices that have kale, beetroot, spinach as their main ingredients, unless of course you are a big fan of these vegetables and you love the earthy taste they offer.

Once you have found a few juices you like then gradually work your way up to having a few juices each week. Then try replacing a meal with a juice and see how you feel about that.

The key to success is to start off small and just introduce juicing to your diet, that way your body won't go into total shock when it gets nothing but juices for a whole 7 days.

If you are already at this point and have been taking in liquid sunlight for a while now, and you are ready to go for seven days on nothing but juice, then congratulations! The key now is to have a peek at some other foods that might give you some grief when you go without them for a long period of time.

Caffeine. Yes, many of us start the day with a morning coffee and the thought of not having that puts us into a frenzy, but the funny thing is, all of the juice fasters I spoke to about this did not actually have any issues with this, so it may not be a big deal for you either.

From my own experience (and I love my morning coffee), I found having a hot lemon water with honey in the morning before I had my juice was sufficient enough to get me through. But, if you have major concerns around this then try replacing one cup of coffee with a herbal tea (not green, as it has caffeine) and see how you go.

The aim is to reduce your reliance on caffeine so that when you fast you don't have to also deal with this withdrawal as well. Please note: reducing caffeine does not mean decaf. The processing involved in taking a natural coffee bean made by mother nature, and turning it into one that doesn't have caffeine makes it extremely hard for your body to process, so it isn't worth drinking. Please don't go down this path thinking this is the way to reduce your intake of caffeine.

Alcohol. If you are like many of us, a nightly/weekly glass of something alcoholic is part of your standard routine (nothing wrong with that). However, if the mere thought of going without any alcohol for seven days has you shaking in your boots, then hmmmm, maybe you need to have a look at that anyway. But, for those that can easily go without, then this is more around managing the period of time you fast. You want to pick a week where you don't have any important social events and where you can fully commit to seven days on juice. If you decide to juice fast for seven days, allow a ten day clearance in your social calendar: one day before and two days after, so ten in total.

Chocolate/Sugar. So, how to go without something sweet? Well, thing is, you will probably find that you won't miss a beat when it comes to sweetness in your diet. Mother Nature is sweet and for most people, they don't have any issues with this, there is plenty of sweetness in fruit and vegetables. In fact, the opposite is probably true you will probably look for something salty/ savoury instead (remember 'real salt', the kind from nature Himalayan Rock Salt or Celtic Sea Salt is totally okay, if not encouraged, when you are fasting).

I would suck on a piece of rock salt (about the size of your little finger nail) or add a tiny bit to water when I felt the need for something salty (too much and you will give yourself a good clean out, so go easy).

So, speaking of which, this leads us to the last item, and no doubt one of the most important

Salt. We all know that our bodies contain a lot of water, (research says between 50-75%). What you might not know is the water contained within our body is salty. Yep, just like the ocean. So, make sure you continue to take in some salt when you fast, again, I am talking good salt here, (Himalayan Rock Salt or Celtic Sea Salt) and it will serve you really well.

Our body uses the sodium (ions) present in salt to perform a variety of essential functions such as maintaining the fluid in our blood cells and transmitting information through our nerves and muscles. It is also used to balance sugar levels in the blood and is vital for absorption of nutrients through our intestinal tract. The body cannot make salt and so we are reliant on food to ensure that we get the required intake.

So, add a good pinch of salt to your juices or suck on it through the day and you will give your body all that it needs!

Go gentle on yourself when you are fasting, or even leading up to one. You don't want to commit to more than you truly believe is possible so just be kind and it will ensure that you have a successful result, each and every time.

"The beginning is the most important part of the work."

~ Plato (Born 427BC)

Plato was Socrates' student who was a philosopher, as well as a mathematician, and he founded the first institution in the western world of higher learning in Athens, Greece.

CHAPTER 4

Getting started

With a juice fast, the first decision is always a very emotional decision, it's the why. The practical stuff around getting a juicer, finding the right time in your calendar or choosing recipes comes in after you've found your why.

Just like any of the big goals in life we undertake, we need to lay the emotional and mental foundation before we begin.

So, how does one begin?

Remember, I am coming from a place of good health, feeling good within my body and choosing to fast as a way to maintain optimum health and to create longevity, so that is my point of reference. Of course, there are heaps of testimonials from all sorts of people who have come to juice fasting because of sickness or because of a diagnosis. If this is your starting point, then join communities and build your belief by hearing from real people, who really did fast and who really did get great results. This is always an easy way to motivate and inspire yourself to do something: take notice of people who have already walked the path before you.

For me, the emotional part of fasting is your WHY and the mental part is your BELIEF. The why is your drive, the thing that pulls you through when/if the going gets tough. Without a big enough why you may find it easy to give up when the body starts to release toxins and you feel a bit average. Without a big enough why you may find you talk yourself out of it at the first sign of feeling hungry, or the minute someone invites you out to dinner.

This is probably why many people only embrace fasting when they have been diagnosed with something and if that diagnosis carries a 'ticking time bomb' (say three months to live), then that is enough of a reason to motivate and ensure commitment right the way through. The will to live is very, very strong and can be a great motivator that will hold focus.

But, what happens when you are coming to this through simple maintenance? You just want to continue to live a great life with all its fineries and you want to do a juice fast so you can continue to maintain optimum health and longevity and appreciate food even more!

The fact you are even reading this book tells me you already have a why. So, this is the part where you get to come clean with yourself. You get to take a deep breath and admit that maybe all is not as you'd prefer. Maybe you have a bit extra around your middle that you'd rather wasn't there. Maybe you have noticed your craving for sugary food or drink. Maybe you have been feeling more tired or lethargic than usual or maybe your internal workings are whispering at you to give them some tender loving care? (Hopefully, they are only whispering - it's a real bitch when they scream!)

Or maybe you have just reached an age where feeling good, having awesome health and looking after your vehicle from the inside out, is more important than the next social outing.

Whatever your reason, find it. Discover your why and let it inform you throughout every shitty moment. Trust me, you won't need it or need to even think about it when you are flying high and feeling like you could climb the tallest mountain, but for those times when your energy wanes and you don't feel crash hot (generally the first three days), you will need a big why to continue to hold your focus and pull you through.

So, we have the why sorted, we now need to build your belief.

This next section is about getting you started in terms of your belief, it's about helping you get from where you are right now to where you want to be - a successful juice faster. All of the practical tools, like what juicer to buy etc. can be found in the chapter called *Juicing Toolkit*, so look to this area for all of the practical things to get your juice fast underway.

I am sure you have come across the saying *"Know Thyself"* the origins of this saying are hard to say but I remember coming across a lovely story about the Delphic Oracle and how this saying was inscribed by the Seven Sages of Greece who challenged all those who came seeking the oracle to *'first seek self-knowledge'*.

To me, this is what juicing gives you – not only knowledge about your body and what it is capable of but it builds a really strong belief and a deep wisdom within you that honestly makes you feel that you can pretty much do anything you set your mind to. I mean to say, if you can go without food for an extended time and survive – seriously, you are on fire my friend and there ain't nuttin' holding you back!!!

So, let's build some belief around juice fasting.

If you haven't fasted before, you might be struggling to believe that you can actually go without food, but if you have managed to start slow and go without food for a day or more, you have already started to build your belief that it is possible.

The key is to start where you are. If you have never gone without a meal in your life, then start adding juices to your diet. When you feel comfortable drinking juices, try replacing one meal with a juice and see how that feels. Then, when you feel comfortable replacing a meal with a juice (and you notice you don't die) push it out to two meals, then a whole day, then try two days etc. Before you know it, seven whole days on nothing but liquid sunlight will be easy!

Another great way to build belief is to tap into people who have already done what you want to do, read books, watch movies, go online and search out other people who already have a really strong belief around this.

A great movie, if you haven't already seen it is *Fat, Sick and Nearly Dead,* by Joe Cross and the sequel *Fat, Sick and Nearly Dead 2.* Joe's first documentary tells the story of his journey to not only clean up his act, but inspire thousands of people right across America to follow his lead. The sequel is filled with testimonials and doctors who have jumped on board the 'juice bus' and achieved amazing results. So, do yourself a favour and purchase his dvds (after all, he is a fellow Aussie and doing really great work, so jump on board).

Personally, I found the best way to build belief is through communities. Join with people who are like-minded. People who have already done what you are about to do and who have achieved great results. For me, I always find juice fasting easiest when you have company, so if you don't have someone physically to fast with, find a virtual friend instead. Whether you know them or not doesn't matter, the fact you have juice fasting in common will unite you. There are a number of communities for juice fasting – here's a couple I have connected with:

Reboot with Joe

Joe Cross has a free online community at http://community.rebootwithjoe.com/

Here you will find discussion forums, recipes you can print, frequently asked questions and videos from real people who have achieved amazing results!

Online Juice Fast

Tyler Tolman, who is the most amazing, funny, wise person I know, has a fantastic online community @ http://tylertolman.com/online-juice-fast.

Here you will find everything from daily rituals, recipes, support groups, exercises, oil pulling, skin cleansing (the list goes on and on) all provided free of charge to help you have the best possible juice fast experience.

I encourage you to sign up to these various online communities and let their belief, their testimonials, and their stories of what they did and how they did it inspire you. Real people, real advice: stuff that works!

When you are connected to other juice fasters you will come to realise (if you haven't already) that juice fasting isn't a weird, new-age, spiritual thing (only done by yogis and Buddhists alike), but rather it's an ancient tool that is now backed by science, and it actually works.

People from all over the world have healed so many illnesses through simply giving their digestive system a break for an extended period.

I encourage you to connect with these online communities and share your story. Even if you are a seasoned faster, you will not only receive a great deal from the stories that are shared, but if you feel inspired to share your story, other people get to learn from your experiences. We all love knowing that we've been able to help another being on their journey and the truth is, we never know when we may need an answer to a question or a kind word to help us on our path and so, do your bit to share your own personal journey and we all get to benefit from your experience.

Now, if you don't feel comfortable fasting by yourself and you don't want to join any of the online communities then look up places that offer 'fasting programs' where you can be guided by experienced practitioners through your fast. Retreats all over the world have programs in place to take you through an extended fast.

Tyler Tolman runs a juice fast program out of Bali and Joe Cross runs his program from Costa Rica, so both of these are definitely worth a check out if you want to get away from your day-to-day life and complete your fast.

Or, if you want to experience a truly amazing program in my home town (which is Melbourne, Australia), then check out *Amarant Retreat* which was founded by a beautiful friend of mine, Dr Hanna Cyncynatus. Amarant rests in 25 acres of magical temperate-rainforest 70km north east of Melbourne and their guided juice fast program called 'Reset your Life' is well worth a look if you want to be inspired and learn a whole heap of great stuff while you are enjoying your fast experience.

So, we've discussed the why and we've hopefully built some belief, now we need to plan our fast.

For me, the best way to prepare for a fast is like preparing for a dinner party with friends and that is with *focused effort and planning.*

With a dinner party the first decision is always to have one. Then you decide on a good time to have it and who you will invite. Once this is sorted, you start to rummage through recipe books to put together a magnificent menu.

Depending on who is coming and how fancy you are making it, you might even try out a few recipes in advance of the big event. From here, it's preparing for the night: food and wine is bought, house is cleaned, glasses are chilled, music is chosen, pre-cooking is done and this is all before the very first person has walked through the door.

So, back to your fast. You've made a decision to do a juice fast, next you need to decide how long you want to fast for. If you decide you want to do seven days then you need to find the best seven days in your schedule so you are not sidelined by having social events interrupt or take you off course during this time. It's also important to decide whether you will start on a weekend or a weekday.

I personally like to start on a weekend, that way the first couple of days (which are generally the toughest) can be spent however you need to spend them - in bed, watching movies, relaxing or whatever - rather than having to do a full day's work on the first day of your fast, which, for some, can be really tough.

So, once you have chosen your time and locked this into your schedule, next thing is to work out which juices you are going to make. If you have chosen to do a seven day juice fast, you will need to make twenty one juices. Whether you want twenty one *different* juices (which is what you will find in the recipe section) or not is up to you. Being a foodie, I like to enjoy different tastes. I get bored with the same flavour over and over, so I mix it up; although I must say in amongst the twenty one juices, I do have some definite favourites (Banana-listic & Gazpacho) which I make a couple of times during the seven days.

The recipe section (further on in the book) gives you the best of the best recipes. These are juices that have been tried and tested by Gary and I, and plenty of other fasters. They have made the grade because of how they taste and what they do within your body and in fact, the order in which they appear has a great significance, so I encourage you to follow the order as well.

*"It is the mark of an educated mind to be able
to entertain a thought without accepting it."
~ Aristotle (384-322 B.C.E.)*

*Aristotle was a Greek philosopher and scientist who taught
Alexander the Great. He was trained first in medicine, and
then in 367 he was sent to Athens to study philosophy with
Plato. He was considered the first genuine scientist in history.*

CHAPTER 5

The first three days

For those of you who may not have done a juice fast before, let me start by saying "the first three days can be a real bitch!" I am sorry, but there really is no other way to express it honestly - the first three days can be tough. Of course, there are exceptions to every rule and if you fall into this category of experiencing an easy ride, then I congratulate you on having what would seem to be a pretty non-toxic system - well done!!!

But, if you are a fairly typical person who lives a fairly typical life, then chances are you will be feeling a tad out of sorts on days one, two and three.

First, your body is going through some pretty major adjustments. Used to digesting on average three meals a day (plus whatever snacks you give it), your body needs to adjust to having all of its food pretty much digested for it. Imagine that, it's probably how your guests feel turning up to your dinner party: they get to just turn up, do small talk, eat, drink and be merry. While you on the other hand, as the host with the most, have been very busy planning, organising, creating, sampling, doing, doing, doing everything to make sure your guests get to kick back and enjoy.

When you prime your body with nothing other than juice to digest, it doesn't actually kick back and do nothing, it actually gets busy because you have freed it up to do so much more.

Check this out:

Your liver - known for having a hand in pretty much every process within the body - gets to offload some of its toxins via the gastrointestinal tract. You may experience some discomfort over your liver area (on the right side of your body just below the ribcage, if you haven't been acquainted yet). If you experience pain or discomfort there, try gently massaging the area with some cold-pressed coconut oil and drinking some lemon juice in warm water to assist the work your liver's doing.

Kidneys - yes, we have two of them and they work hard to purify our blood and eliminate waste, so they will love you for flushing them out with liquid sunlight. Its okay if you run to the toilet a lot in the first few days as your body adjusts to your new diet and toxins are removed from your bloodstream, so just go with it. Your kidneys are thanking you for giving them a flush and they will respond in kind when you get back to normal eating. Remember to continue to drink plenty of water during your fast (even though you are drinking juice) as this will help to carry the toxins out.

Your lungs - yes, the lungs get to eliminate all of that toxic pollution you have taken in and any other toxins that may have been bundled up and pushed into the lung cavity so it could be coughed up and out. Remember, every organ is engaged in an internal spring clean during your fast so allow yourself some space to breathe through this time. Don't get upset with yourself if you feel out of breath or tired, let your body rest. To help with this, try putting a couple of drops of Peppermint Essential Oil on the palm of your hand and then rubbing your two hands together (vigorously) and then when you have them nice and warm, cup them around your nose and breathe in deeply and let the Peppermint Oil work its magic on your respiratory system.

Your stomach - ahhh, the one that is the hardest working of all. Our digestive system runs from our mouth through our stomach, into our small intestines and colon, and exits via our back door. When you start to detox you may feel a bit of nausea as you change your diet and, of course, as your gastrointestinal tract also gets an opportunity to eliminate toxins. Ginger tea helps alleviate this, so just take it easy and take in what feels right during this time, don't push yourself. If you are not up for a juice, don't have it. Just drink plenty of water. Often nausea is a result of dehydration so make sure you keep the water intake up, and know that this will pass.

Your skin - given it is the largest organ in your body (yes, it is an organ!) it is quite common to notice pimples, rashes or other lesions appearing during your juice fast. This is a great sign that your body is pushing toxins to the surface so don't be alarmed and please don't put anything unnatural onto your skin, thinking you are helping the healing process. (The key to knowing whether something is natural or not, is; can you eat it?)

If you want to assist the healing process, do some skin brushing (Gwasha) which not only feels totally amazing, but it helps remove the toxins from your body.

To make the Gwasha mix you need some triple distilled vodka and some bicarb soda. Quite simply, you make a paste using vodka and bicarb soda (make sure the bicarb soda is food grade and aluminium free) and gently scrub your body with the paste. Do this each morning before you shower, then have your shower. To super-enhance this process, spend some time in the sun afterwards and your skin will glow like never before and the Vitamin D you take into each of your cells after such a cleanse is truly beneficial. Your body will thank you for it!

The tongue - Most people I know experience a coated tongue whenever they do a juice fast. The more coated it is, the more toxins are being released. The tongue is an indicator of what is happening internally, especially along the gastrointestinal tract. If you want to help this process, give oil pulling a go: it's fantastic! Basically, every morning before you drink anything or clean your teeth you place about a tablespoon of cold pressed organic coconut oil into your mouth (no swallowing) and swish it around for about 20 minutes.

As you swish, the coconut oil is literally pulling toxins out of your body. After about 20 minutes the oil will be quite thick and white - spit it out (never swallow this - it is full of toxins!!!). What I have also noticed is this process also clears all sorts of conditions, from yellowing teeth to acne to deep internal issues. It's an ancient Indian health ritual and if you do a search on it online you will be amazed at the results people have achieved from doing it every day.

Apart from everything I have mentioned above going on within your body, you may also experience general symptoms to some degree. Mild headaches are quite common. The dull, achy types are the norm. The pain relates to toxins being dumped into the bloodstream and circulated throughout the body and brain before elimination. Make sure you keep hydrated with lots of water to shift the headache. The key to getting rid of a headache is to flood your system with water, drink one litre all at once (no sipping it) and then wait fifteen minutes and you may just find your headache has gone. Another tip is to drink some Organic Cherry Juice as cherries are a natural pain reliever, so you might find this helpful as well.

Weakness or lethargy is common as well. Your body is focused on cleaning and diverts energy internally instead of for motion and strength. So, achy muscles and flu-like symptoms may appear as toxins work their way out of your system. A massage by a caring friend/partner or a professional will greatly help this process and help you to feel a bit more relaxed and peaceful.

You may also notice you feel cold during your fast. This is due to your body temperature decreasing as you decrease your calorie intake. If you find yourself in need of some warmth, ginger tea is a great herbal tea to warm you up from the inside, so make sure you have some fresh ginger on hand (or herbal teabags). Or alternatively, if you have access to a bath, then nothing beats a hot bath to which you've added some Himalayan Rock Salt and some bubble bath (made from natural ingredients, of course). Remember to put on some soft, relaxing music, light some candles and allow all of your senses to be pampered - you deserve it!

With all of what you have just read you may not even want to start a juice fast now and I completely understand. But, remember just fasting on juice for three days will give your immune system such a boost that it is well worth going through any discomfort for this short period. I mean to say, what's a weekend out of your life? Your body will take so much from just three days, where you don't have to digest food that you will easily build to seven days in no time. I think science is actually catching up to this fact now and if you search online for what the benefits of just doing a three day juice fast are, you might be surprised to find all sorts of great medical studies in support of this. But ultimately, it comes down to your why: is it for health reasons, maintenance, or weight loss? Is it to rid, repair and rejuvenate your body? Or, is it to simply give it a go and prove to yourself that you can? Whatever the reason for wanting to do it, make sure you keep your why front of mind and it will pull you through if/when the going gets tough.

Trust your body and know that every cell loves you and is actually working for you. The pain you are feeling is a sure sign that the fast is effective and the body is cleaning itself of all of the old, hidden and stored toxins. This reaction is temporary, trust me. It sucks, I know, but it is temporary and if you keep going until the fourth day, you will be pleasantly, if not miraculously, surprised.

So, on that note – let me give you a little taste of what is to come on day four.

Day four is fantastic for most people. Gone is the dull, achy head and feeling out of sorts. Most people wake up with a new lease on life. Their energy stores have gone through the roof, they feel alive, awake and refreshed. They have clarity like never before and their focus is as sharp as an eagle's vision.

Yes, day four is tremendous, you feel like you have a new lease on life and your innards feel better than ever before. So, trust me, it is seriously worth getting to this day, for on this day you truly know that you have made it, even though, if you are doing a seven day fast, you still have a few days to go. This is the turning point where you can pat yourself on the back and congratulate yourself for pushing through when you might have wanted to give up. For most people it's smooth sailing from here on end, so get to this day and know that it's all feel good from here!

"We are not rich by what we possess, but by what we can do without."

~ *Immanuel Kant (1724 – 1804)*

Immanuel Kant was a German philosopher who studied philosophy, mathematics and physics. His individual study of knowledge examined the basis of human knowledge and its limits.

CHAPTER 6

Juicing toolkit

To start off, if you are going to juice, you need a juicer. Now, before you rush off and purchase the most expensive or least expensive juicer on the market, here are a few things you might like to consider. Not all juicers (and not all juices) are created equal.

As you will discover, there are tonnes of different juicers on the market. And they all claim to be the bee's knees when it comes to juicing fruit and vegetables. So before you part with your cash, here are some things that are helpful to know.

No 1. The quality of juice varies from machine to machine!

Yes, hard to believe I know, but the quality of juice your juicer spits out is pretty high on the things to consider list. Trust me, you want to know that your body is getting the absolute maximum out of every apple crushed, every carrot masticated and every bit of kale squeezed!

No 2. It makes a difference when your juicer is easy to clean.

Not everyone is that fussed when it comes to how easy your juicer is to clean, but when you are juicing three times a day for seven days, you want something that makes the job a little easier, so take this into consideration when you go looking at juicers - you will be thankful you did!

No 3. Peace and quiet is not overrated!

Some juicers sound like a jet engine starting up, which is all well and good if you are into jet engines, but not if you are up early to get your juices ready before work and you wake your entire household up with the noise coming from your juicer. We found this one an important factor for us, so look for juicers that keep the peace.

No 4. Cold Press vs Centrifugal - who wins?

Well, here's where the jury rests. We personally like cold press juicers. Why? Because, not only do you get more juice (which is very important if you are living off this stuff for a week) but, the juice you get is super high quality and tastes way better. The other thing you will notice is the colour of juice from a cold press juicer is just gorgeous (bright, vivid and pretty much just as liquid sunshine should be!) whereas often the juice from a centrifuge juicer is murky/brown in colour. The juice out of a centrifuge juicer is watery whereas the juice out of a cold pressed juicer is not, it an enzyme rich juice. With a cold press juicer the fruit and veg is masticated by a very slow spinning ball – so you get a much denser (filled with all the good stuff) juice!

But, there are plenty of people who say that a centrifuge juicer is by far the best, which is a juicer that has spinning blades.

What we do know is the juice made out of a centrifugal juicer will oxidise much faster (within 24 hours), so you won't be able to store it for long, whereas a juice made out of a cold press juicer can be stored in an airtight glass container for up to 48 hours without losing any nutritional qualities. I don't know about you, but we really enjoy making our juices in advance and having them at the ready for when we are working, so a cold press juicer wins hands down from that point of view.

We actually have both types of juicers so I actually speak from experience and in my opinion, the cold press juicer wins hands down.

As for what brand of juicer to buy. We love Kuvings Cold Press Juicer, it truly is the best and it ticks all of the boxes I mentioned before. It is quiet, easy to clean and the juice is nutrient rich.

But at the end of the day, buy what feels right for you, and what you can afford – at least you are juicing, which is the number one most important thing. Let yourself start somewhere and by doing that, you will build your awareness and become wise in the process.

No 5. What about fruit juices – don't they contain loads of sugar?

I ask you, have you ever cut open a piece of fruit and seen sugar? No, you haven't, have you? So, the simple answer is, fruit does not contain sugar.

The scientific answer is: the sweetness in fruit is called fructose which is a simple sugar that occurs *naturally* in foods. It gives fruits their sweet taste. In a normally healthy person, the natural sugar in fruits is easily assimilated and digested (unlike white, processed table sugar which is toxic and addictive to the body). Fruit juices generally have a low glycemic index (GI), which means that it doesn't make the glucose level in the blood rise as fast and as high as a high GI food.

No 6. A juicer is not a blender and vice versa.

People often confuse a blender with a juicer and vice versa. Juicing is the method of extracting juice, and only juice, from fruits or vegetables. All of the pulp and fibre is removed, which allows the nutrients to assimilate very quickly into your body and bloodstream; this gives your immune system an immediate boost and feeds your cells with quick, healing nutrition.

A blender blends the fruit and vegetables you put into it so you get a smooth drink (smoothie). Smoothies are generally thick and creamy in texture, whilst a juice is watery and thin. Smoothies are great to have when you want to get a big hit of fruit and veg, (greens for instance) and most kids love them.

No 7. Organic vs Non-Organic

Of course, using organic fruit and vegetables is ideal, not only to support this industry but to get the best of the best, however it is not mandatory. The key is to make sure you give your non-organic produce a little wash in organic, cold-pressed Apple Cider Vinegar (about ¼ cup to a sink full of water) before you eat it. This simple wash will remove any chemicals on the surface of the produce and we've found all of our produce stays fresh for much longer.

I guess the most important thing is to make sure you use fruit and vegetables that are in season (not produce that has been in cold storage for months/years). So, build your recipes around that.

Worth mentioning here is that all of the recipes within this book have been created in winter time so, the produce is seasonal to winter – if you are doing your fast in summer, have a look at what recipes suit the produce available during this time (ie: Minty Melon, Cabala, Pineapple Punch) and go from there.

"You have to make the rules, not follow them."
~ Sir Isaac Newton (1643 – 1727)

Sir Isaac Newton is widely recognised as one of the most influential scientists of all time and as a key figure in the scientific revolution. He was an English physicist and mathematician who was most famous for his law of gravitation.

CHAPTER 7

Juice recipes

Here's where all the fun begins. The recipe section that tells you what and how much you need to buy to enjoy three juice meals a day for seven days.

Each recipe makes one litre of juice and has been through a rigorous testing process, which basically means we made it, tried it and if it didn't taste good to us, then it didn't make the grade. We also gave these recipes to friends and other fellow juicers to try and if any of them came back saying they didn't like something, then we made changes to make sure we had a good variety and above all, tasted great!

The other thing to note is, this book was written over the winter time, which is why the juices are based on fruit and vegetables that are seasonal to winter – if you are juice fasting in summer, then I encourage you to head online and find juice recipes for this time of year that you can use.

Of course, this is only a guide – truly, you can jump online and search for juice recipes and find gazillions of them – so, if you don't like the sound of these, then find your own or have fun making up your own recipes based on what you like.

We have also put together a couple of helpful tools to help you with your juice fast:

A Foodies Guide Weekly Planner, which is basically all twenty one juices on one page which you can print out as an easy reference guide to making each juice. We stuck this on our fridge and used it as a guide for what fruit and veg was needed for each juice. The 'Weekly Planner' is available on my website: www.juliannedowse.com

A Foodies Guide Shopping List, which is also available on my website, is an easy to use spreadsheet that you can download, plug in all of your juice ingredients and get a total of which ingredients to buy. Some people like to shop as they go along, but we find that buying the whole seven days' ingredients at once helps us stick to the fast. We found that it worked for us to buy everything at once, and besides, the looks on the faces of the people who serve you when you have that much of 'nature's health' in your trolley is priceless!

Each recipe makes 1 litre of juice which is pretty much what you need for each meal. However, everyone is different so please adjust, up or down as you need.

Juice Recipes

1. **Pineapple Punch**

   – bursting with sunshine and goodness, sweet and juicy!

   2 carrots

   2 oranges peeled

   1/2 pineapple

   1/2 lime skin removed

2. **PLP**

   – smooth on the taste buds, sweet and cleansing

   4 pears

   1/2 lemon

   1 bunch parsley

3. **Gazpacho**

   – savoury and delicious, just like cold tomato soup

   4 tomatoes

   1 capsicum

   3 celery stalks

   ¼ onion

   1 cucumber

   1 clove garlic

   1 lime skin removed

4. **Minty Melon**

   – sweet, fresh and cooling for the body

   1/2 watermelon

   1 bunch mint

5. **The Hydrator**

   – sweet with a bitey tang

   2 carrots

   4 oranges peeled

   4 red apples

   1 bunch mint

   1 grapefruit

   3 celery stalks

6. **Vitality**

   – savoury and light, giving a delicious hit of goodness!

   2 carrots

   3 handfuls kale

   1 green apple

   1 red apple

   1/2 cucumber

   4 celery stalks

   1 bunch parsley

   500ml coconut water

7. **Pineapple Tonic**

   – sweet, lip smacking zinger

   1 grapefruit

   1/2 pineapple

   1 knob ginger

   500ml coconut water

8. **PCK**

   – a sweet surprise

   2 carrots

   3 celery stalks

   3 kale handfuls

   2 kiwi

   4 pears

   1 bunch parsley

9. **Banana-listic**

   – a sweet, decadent and scrumptious cocktail

   2 bananas

   2 young coconuts, flesh and water

   * add extra coconut water as needed

10. **Oh IC**

– sweet with a hint of tang

4 carrots

4 oranges peeled

2 handfuls of spinach

11. **Apple-aide**

– sweet, fresh and light

4 green apples

1 bok choy

1 cucumber

1 lemon

12. **Thermal Tonic**

– savoury with a dash of spice that is warming for the body

8 radishes

1/2 beetroot

10 carrots

2 cucumber

1 lemon

1 knob ginger

13. **OB1**

- deliciously different with a hint of sweet

1 broccoli head

4 oranges peeled

4 apples

1 knob of ginger

14. **Green Machine**

– a sweet and smooth green goddess

4 celery stalks

4 green apples

3 handfuls kale

2 kiwis

250ml coconut water

15. **Tomato Tonic**

- savoury with a hint of spice

4 tomatoes

2 punnets cherry tomatoes

4 celery stalks

1/2 beetroot

1 bunch basil

1 clove garlic

1 lemon

16. **Smooth Operator**

- heavenly sweet and delicious

2 kiwis

4 oranges peeled

2 pears

1/2 pineapple

1/2 lime

17. **ABC**

- fresh and light with a hint of sweetness

4 yellow apples

1 head of broccoli

1/2 cucumber

250ml coconut water

18. **Pink Lady**

– sweet, spicy, wholesome goodness

5 red apples

1/2 beetroot

1/2 lemon

1 knob of ginger

250ml coconut water

19. **Sweet Ginger**

– sweet and bitey

4 carrots

1 pineapple

1 lemon

1 knob of ginger

20. **Lean Green**

– sweet, fresh and inviting

3 green apples

1 cucumber

1/2 honey dew melon

21. **C.A.B.A.L.A**

– medicinal magic in liquid form (blessings to Don Toman)

4 carrots (C)

1 green apple (A)

1/2 beetroot (B)

1 red apple (A)

1/2 lemon (L)

1 yellow apple (A)

*If you don't have different colour apples, that's cool - just use one colour

"Big results require big ambitions."
        ~ Heraclitus (535BC – 475BC)

*Heraclitus was a pre-Socratic Greek philosopher who
believed in the unity of opposites, stating that "the
path up and down are one and the same."*

CHAPTER 8

Juicy bits

Fasting is not *just* about taking in liquid sunlight for an extended period, any type of fasting (abstinence), whether that be from meat, junk food, coffee, alcohol, sugar, cigarettes or just food in general, does one of two things:

1. It changes you.
2. You have to practice mindfulness in order to be successful at it.

So, how does it change you and what is mindfulness?

Well, change begins from the inside out. The saying about 'being the change you wish to see in the world' is about that, change begins firstly on the inside.

So, not only is our body going to feel clean (which is no doubt different from what we are used to) there will be subtle changes to how you view the world and your life. You simply can't help but be changed from a juice fasting experience - the key is to go with the change and don't resist it or beat yourself up for thinking or feeling different as a result.

Mindfulness means we are being conscious of our thoughts, we are aware. So, practicing mindfulness is when we turn our attention to what it is we are actually doing, rather than operating on auto-pilot.

Most things we do on a regular basis are pretty automatic: we don't have to think too much about doing them, we just do them habitually, like smoking, eating, drinking, craving sugar, having our morning coffee etc. We do these mostly without thinking, it's just what we do.

For instance, let's take a morning coffee (for us coffee drinkers), if you are not a coffee drinker, insert something else you do on a regular basis without thinking. So, back to our coffee - usually your mind will only kick into gear if you *don't* have it, rather than when you do. Your mind is simply running a program (which you have created, I might add) that says 'it's morning and that equals coffee'.

But what if once a week on a Wednesday, you decided to replace your morning coffee with a juice? You might find it easy to remember the first time you do it, but the second, third and probably fourth time you might have to remind yourself that you are only having a juice on Wednesdays, and not a coffee, until you are unconsciously competent - which means, you are on auto-pilot.

The thing is, our 'normal' is only our normal because we say it is. All of the things we do on a regular basis end up becoming comfortable (our comfort zone), and when we become comfortable in anything, it takes a *change of mind* (which leads to a change in action) to create a different result. Once a neural pathway has been established in our brain, it takes a conscious change, a change in our thinking, to establish a new pathway - which in turn, leads to a new 'normal'.

In recent years, we have learned that the brain is plastic, which effectively means it can be moulded, shaped and coerced down all sorts of paths to believe what we want it to believe - and not just be stuck with the program we have either been given, or which we have created unconsciously.

So when you do a juice fast, a big part of the challenge is to do with your thoughts. Sure, don't get me wrong, the body goes through a whole heap of great stuff: digestive processes change, our elimination cycle shifts, inflammation in our body is reduced, lungs clear out excess mucous, tubes are cleaned up, blockages are removed, tumours are dissolved and pretty much the 'clean-up crew' hits the streets and does a magnificent job of getting rid of all of the stuff our body doesn't need.

But what you might not realise is that you actually get to take control of your mind. You get to practice mindfulness. Now to me this is the most important thing in the world, and by far the biggest benefit from completing an extended fast of seven days.

Why, you ask...

Well, the thing is...LIFE HAPPENS!

And what I mean by that is, we truly can't control life.

Now I am sure we all get that and also understand that we can only ever control how we react to life, to things that happen to us.

For instance, I couldn't control (as much as I would have loved to) the death of my mother. As much as I would give anything to still have her around today, it was out of my control because I didn't know what I didn't know and we didn't have the information or understanding of how to really treat what was going on for her. And so, she suffered horribly for over six months and when she eventually died we were all just faceless strangers in the hospital room; the drugs had taken her mind and spirit long ago and sadly her body was just taking its time catching up.

So, in that instance what I could control is how I reacted to her death. Rather than it be a crippling trauma that took me a long time to get through (or never get through), I had the choice of how I thought about it. With a big heart full of love and loads of beautiful memories from spending over thirty years with her in my life, I focused all of my energy on all the good stuff and it made me smile and feel happy inside. And, what that did was allowed me to get on with my life in a really positive, healthy way and to this day, whenever I think of my beautiful mother (pretty much every day) I smile and feel love and that is a true blessing.

Another example of turning a negative situation into a positive experience was when my work contract wasn't extended (even though I had worked in the same organisation for a very long time). At the time, with a mortgage and loans to pay for, I was very reliant on having a wage and so this could have been a really, really stressful time, but focusing my energy towards what I wanted (a better job with more money) allowed me to see the opportunities that were being presented instead of being too caught up in 'woe is me energy' that would have surely had me unemployed for a long time. Instead, I saw it as an opportunity to make some changes and so by reacting well to the change, not only did I find some new work really quickly, I carved out a whole new career which led to me earning much more money than ever before.

You might think all of this is totally unrelated, but this is actually where juice fasting stands in a league of its own.

When you decide to stop eating and take into your body nothing but juice, your mind goes a little crazy. It doesn't quite get that food doesn't actually keep you alive and it thinks that without food you are simply going to die. Armed with those thoughts, your body responds accordingly. You may get the shakes, you may feel dizzy, you may have no energy, you might even have little panic attacks, basically, your mind will do whatever it needs to do in order to get you to eat and stay alive.

And I must say if you are not armed with good information about what is happening to your body, you will probably go straight back to eating (or smoking, or whatever it is you are trying to change).

But if you know that people have successfully fasted for years and years, for extensive periods of time, you then understand that your mind is just programmed with old, out of date information and it just needs a new program. So, give it one and you will be amazed at what you can achieve.

The key here is belief. You can't succeed in life without belief, you must believe you can do something, believe in yourself, and make the rules so you win. You simply can do anything you set for yourself if you truly believe it is possible.

Long before I was into any of this healthy stuff, I used to physically shake if I had gone past a mealtime, my body would ache for food and I would actually get quite irritable. God help anyone who tried to come between me and my food back then.

Today, I am very comfortable going without food for long periods of time and my body doesn't falter. The internal strength and confidence as a result of all of the work I have done is priceless, absolutely priceless.

So if nothing else, fast for the simple fact you will take control of the 'monkey mind', cos who knows when you will need to draw upon that reserve of strength to overcome a 'life situation' - and trust me, you and those you will want to support, will be better for it.

"Have the courage to use your own reasons.
That is the motto of enlightenment"
~ Immanuel Kant (1724 – 1804)

Immanuel Kant was a German philosopher who studied philosophy,
mathematics and physics. His individual study of knowledge
examined the basis of human knowledge and its limits.

CHAPTER 9

Frequently asked questions

Q. Can I drink coffee/tea/alcohol/soft drinks during my juice fast?

No - coffee, tea, alcohol or soft drinks in any form is allowed. However, herbal teas (peppermint, chamomile, ginger etc) are all good. Keep in mind that Green Tea contains caffeine so you will need to avoid it. Try lemon in hot water if you want something hot and soothing—this is also fantastic for the liver and to help detox add a spoon of raw honey and you have a very yummy drink.

Q. Can I take painkillers for my headache?

Well, of course you can - however it is best not to if you can manage it. Headaches are a sure sign that your body is working hard to eliminate toxins, so giving it another toxin (by way of a painkiller) doesn't help. Try drinking one litre of water, straight up – no sipping, no breaks – just flood your system with water. Your brain (and bowels surprisingly enough) will love you for it. Or, another thing I have tried that works is putting some peppermint oil into a foot bath and giving yourself a lovely foot massage (or better still, ask someone else to) - often this will help drag the energy away from your head and release the headache. I also find that organic cold pressed cherry juice (which is a natural aspirin) works too.

Q. I would like to fast for general maintenance, but I am not overweight, will I lose weight?

In my experience, those who have weight to lose, do, and those who don't, don't. If you haven't anything to lose, you might find that you clean up in certain areas - around your face, arms, legs, neck - places that don't hold a lot of weight but all good areas that lighten up after a juice fast. You'll be surprised how much padding you carry - particularly around your face - and be pleasantly surprised with your new vibrant and youthful look!

Q. Can I smoke during a juice fast?

Well, the aim of a juice fast is to give your body a break, so continuing to smoke and introduce toxins into your body draws the energy of your body to that, rather than focusing on what you wanted it to do which was to repair, rejuvenate and give it a much needed rest! What we have found from the smokers who have juice fasted was that they actually didn't crave a smoke during their fast, so give it a go, you might be pleasantly surprised.

Q. What about fruit juices – don't they contain loads of sugar?

Absolutely not. The sweetness in fruit is called fructose which is a simple sugar that occurs naturally in foods. It gives fruit their sweet taste. In a normally healthy person, the natural sugar in fruits is easily assimilated and digested, unlike table sugar which is toxic to the body. Fruit juices generally have a low glycemic index (GI), which means that it doesn't make the glucose level in the blood rise as fast and as high as a high GI food. So, real fruit juice – the kind you juice yourself or get from a reputable juice company is great!

"Fasting is the greatest remedy, the physician within"

~ Paracelsus (1493 - 1541)

Paracelsus was sixteen when he entered the University at Basle to study alchemy, surgery, and medicine. He was known as the most original medical thinker of the sixteenth century.

CHAPTER 10

Breakfast

No, not breakfast, although that's what breakfast is actually about, it's about breaking your fast. When you have gone without food for an extended period and your digestive system hasn't had to digest for a little while, you will want to introduce food really slowly to ensure you don't undo all of the great work you have just done.

I mean to say who wants to feel awful when you have just spent a whole heap of time feeling great, or if you haven't managed to get to that great space, at least you know that your body has got benefit from what you have accomplished, and so the very last thing you want to do is jump straight back into loading your body with things that are hard to process; meat, sugars, caffeine, alcohol, pasta, rice etc.

The way to break a fast is to do it slowly. When you wake up on day one after a seven day juice fast, think about giving your body some fruit, maybe an apple and some strawberries (or whatever you have left over from your fast). Make a fruit salad and enjoy this for breakfast with a juice. Then for lunch, maybe have a raw salad that has been sprinkled with good olive oil, lemon juice and real salt, again, add a juice to your afternoon and then have a nice light soup for dinner. The key is to keep it light. Fresh, light and easy on your digestive system.

Trust me, your body will be the indicator of whether you have broken your fast well or not. If you start feeling detox symptoms - heavy head, nausea, feeling bloated - then, slow down. Get some water in and take your time to resume normal eating. If you give all of your systems a chance to come back online, you will be thankful you did.

On the second day, start to introduce some old favourites - coffee, tea, bread - but just go gentle and listen to your body, it will tell you what you need and what you don't.

Another thing you might notice is it takes a few days for your bowels to kick back into gear. Allow the transition to happen, have some prunes or Senna tea or grated apple to help speed up the process if you need to, but know that your internal organs are just adjusting to having to come back to work after being on an extended break. I am sure we can all relate to what that feels like when we return from vacation and go back to work, so go slowly, be patient and trust your body to do what it needs to do.

Now, if you need a little help to get your bowels moving, either at the end of your fast or even during - try doing an enema. They are really simple to do, actually very relaxing and your body just loves it. Here's a real quick guide to help you get started:

Here's what you need:

- Surgical Enema Kit (buy online or at your local pharmacy)

- Coconut Oil
- Real salt (Celtic Sea Salt or Himalayan Rock Salt)
- Music, pillow, towel and maybe some candles (whatever creates a nice space for you)

With enema kit in hand, head to your bathroom. On the way, grab a pillow for your head and a towel to lay on and something to listen to (soft, gentle music).

Next – place some coconut oil around your anus and on the enema tube (I always check that I have the 'tube lock' on at this point, otherwise when you fill the canister up with warm salt water the water will come rushing straight out – yes, already been stung by that one once!!).

Find a place where you can lie down comfortably (well, as comfortably as one can get with a small tube inserted very gently up you know what). Lay your towel down and put your pillow on the floor for your head.

Grab your enema canister and sprinkle some salt into it and fill with warm water (not hot!!!). Most enema kits have a little hook to hang it on the towel rail with, but I just stand it on the bathroom bench – works for me.

Get yourself into position with the tube dangling down next to you. Reach down and grab the end of the tube and gently insert and then unclip the 'tube lock' and let the water flow in.

At this point, you can lift up your hips to flow the water around more, or massage your stomach area to move it through. Once all the water is in, remove the tube and enjoy letting it flow through your system. Now, everyone is different, so if you can't take the whole canister full of water into your system, then that's okay – just take in what you can. Over time, you will be able to do it easy I am sure. Now just lie there and wait until you feel the urge to go and when that happens, jump up and let nature do the rest. Another way to help everything flow out much easier is to sit on the toilet with your feet on a small step so your legs form a ninety degree angle.

If you find yourself laying on the ground for ages and you don't feel you have the urge – then get up and go about your day, sometimes just being upright helps flow it all through and out the door (so to speak) very quickly.

What I notice is, I always feel great after an enema. Whether I do it because I am fasting or just because I am feeling a bit out of sorts – enemas' are a great tool to have at your disposal. I use them at the onset of a sniffle, if I ever have an upset tummy or if I feel bloated, but pretty much they can be used for all sorts of complaints (from headaches to insomnia). They are a must for your medicine cupboard. You can even buy travel enema kits which is awesome to have as part of your luggage when you travel overseas.

The key is to not be scared. Enema's are an ancient healing tool and should be used often, not just when we are sick. Tyler Tolman has a great YouTube video that you can watch (no, he doesn't actually do one live), but he does take you through how he does it and how easy they are to do – so, make sure you go online and check that out!

"Let him that would move the world first move himself."
          ~ Socrates (circa 470 BC – 399 BC)

Socrates was a classical Greek (Athenian) philosopher who is credited as one of the founders of Western philosophy. Socrates' wisdom was limited to an awareness of his own ignorance, he always claimed he 'knew nothing'. Socrates invited others to concentrate on friendships and a sense of true community as the best way for people to grow together as a populace.

CHAPTER 11

Faster stories

Before you try anything for the first time, it always pays to follow in the footsteps of those who have gone before you. People who have done what you want to do, who have succeeded and who have some wisdom to share based on their own experience.

And so, in their own words, here are some juice fasting experiences for your reading pleasure.

"Day One - So far so good, 8.30 am and I have not cried over lack of food yet, winning!! Have been to the gym for just a light 30 minutes swim to get the muscles moving and now am on to the first juice, um, YUM!! Give the Pineapple Punch a big thumbs up.

Half way through lunch juice, not as good as breakfast juice, I got a little excited when adding the parsley, but the facial expressions are giving everyone at work something to laugh at. Got half way through lunch juice and have realised that I have not had any water yet. Time to stop with the juice and start on the water, woo hoo!! Everyone ate their lunch down stairs which was chips and hamburgers and .... No one died, so far proud of myself, pat on the back and a smile on my face, 19 hours without food, 485 000 to go!!

Day Four - That little man in my head got me, I had a salad for lunch raw salad, no dressing, but this would now conclude the end of my juice fast. However 3 and a half days and proud of myself for getting that far."

~ Leah, 32

"I lost 5kg, gave up smoking for 5wks. I had an amazing support team and am juicing 3-7 days each month now and feeling great!!"

~ Fiona, 49

"Really enjoyed it, was surprised at how you never felt hungry and had heaps of energy."

~ George, 43

"I found I did not miss anything except walnuts and sultanas."

~ Lorraine, 65

"I don't think it had much impact on me. Lost 2 kilos and managed to keep off 1.5kilos. Though I am more conscious now on what I eat. Try to stay healthy and eat less fatty/processed food."

~ Trang, 37

"First time I fast a full week & I didn't think I can do that at first. The variety of juice recipes really help & doing in a group of friends or colleague to boost motivation."

~ Carly, 32

"Was excited by what the outcomes might be after doing the fast / detox i.e. feeling healthier, fresher, more alive, weight loss and experiencing something different to what I've tried in the past. Followed the preparation for 2 days prior to starting in earnest and I think this helped a lot. Prepared the body and its functions for the upcoming week to some extent and started the week feeling well. After starting the detox in earnest the first day is a breeze and it went very quickly without any side effects. Day 2 and 3 were different, experience a dull headache through the 48 hours and added more water and lemon to the schedule. Pretty much stuck to my exercise routine (swimming 2-3km each day) but had a break on Wednesday to give the body a break. By day 4 I started to come good, headache gone, taste was changing and noticed the swimming had picked up as well. Day 5 was last one at work with the rest of the crew and was a sort of celebration for getting this far and we each treated with favourite juice. Day 6 & 7 at home was great, up early, did lots of things at home and really didn't notice not eating. Coming off the detox was good as I followed Tyler's tips and did it slowly without any side effects. Lost 6.6kgs, 4cm off the waist, 2cm around the chest and a few off the legs. Feel great and the after affects have been great. Most of our team have continued with some of the principles and we have started fasting

1 day a week and will build to 2 days after a month. Having lots of support and enthusiasm during this period, was truly inspiring!"

~ Andrew, 53

"It was a great experience and more satisfying that I ever thought it would be, at the end it felt a lot easier than I thought it would. The best part is that I have subtly changed the way I eat and kept off the weight without dramatically changing my lifestyle."

~ Sam, 38

"I decided to do the juice fast because I really didn't think I could! My diet's pretty good already, so the challenge was more of a mental one for me. I had extra weight that I was happy to lose too, but it wasn't my main focus.

I'm so pleased to report that actually, fasting for seven days was MUCH easier than I thought it would be! Julianne's juice recipes are delicious, and I was never hungry, which was a huge bonus. There were one or two moments when I thought 'that's it, I have had enough of this', but I allowed myself a few moments of fantasy, and then reminded myself of my 'why'. And hooray, I did it! I felt so much cleaner and leaner at the end of the seven days, and noticed that my clothes were fitting so much better.

I didn't incorporate enough of my new-found love of and respect for the benefits of juicing after those seven days, and so am now on Day Six of another fast, which is going really well.

I've created a plan for how to include juice into my life from here on, and a new 'why' to enjoy that 'clean, lean' feeling every day. Thanks so much for the inspiration, the wisdom and the fantastic juices, Julianne!"

~ Caroline, 50

"Don't judge each day by the harvest you reap but by the seeds that you plant."
~ Robert Louis Stevenson (1850 - 1894)

Robert Louis Stevenson, a 19th century Scottish writer who most treasured works include; Treasure Island, Kidnapped, and Strange Case of Dr. Jekyll and Mr. Hyde

CHAPTER 12

Pay it forward

Here's where you get to support someone else on their juice fast journey, because quite naturally, once you have completed your very first juice fast, you will be an expert in this field and people will ask you all sorts of crazy questions.

You could just hand them this book and tell them to do what you have done - read the book, get inspired and then do the fast - or, you could be their juice coach and help them along, which is way more fun and more inspiring for the person undertaking juice fasting for the very first time.

So point them in the right direction, guide them, inspire them and above all else, tell them your truth. Tell them why you did it, what results you achieved, what sucked and what you loved. Let them be inspired by your discipline and commitment to do something that most people think they can't. And, if you find yourself questioning whether to share your journey or not, remember this little story.

"Once a man was walking along a beach. The sun was shining and it was a beautiful day. Off in the distance he could see a person going back and forth between the surf's edge and the beach. Back and forth this person went. As the man approached he could see that there were hundreds of starfish stranded on the sand as the result of the natural action of the tide.

The man was struck by the apparent futility of the task. There were far too many starfish. Many of them were sure to perish. As he approached, the person continued the task of picking up starfish one by one and throwing them into the surf.

As he came up to the young man he said, "You must be crazy. There are thousands of miles of beach covered with starfish. You can't possibly make a difference." The young man looked at him. He then stooped down and picked up one more starfish and threw it back into the ocean. He turned back to the man and said, "It made a difference to that one!"

~ unknown

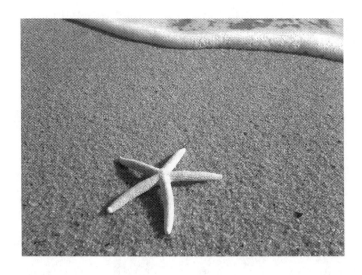

I congratulate you on everything you are about to undertake and my wish for you is that you feel empowered to give it a go and be a beacon of light for others. And, when they say to you (and they will) "Oh my God, I could never do a juice fast I love my food too much", simply give them this book and say "yeah, that's what I used to think to!"

> "Join the self-care revolution,
> Let food be your medicine,
> And fasting be thy healer."
> ~ Gary Dowse

In gratitude

This book could not have come into being without…

Dorothy.

For all of who you were and what you taught me, consciously and unconsciously, I will be forever grateful for all of it. Your light continues to inspire me. Thanks Ma, I love you.

Gary.

My beautiful husband, I love you more than words can say. OMG, who would have thought this would be my first book? That's just too funny! Thank you for believing in me, for keeping me focused and mostly, for sharing your love and wisdom throughout the journey. Yep, this is just the beginning! I love the ancient wisdom that we are surrounding ourselves with and bringing through to help others. I love how we are using it to guide and inform us to create all of what we are creating and I look forward to many more lifetimes together!

Caroline.

The *Secret* bought us together, but it's no secret that we have been together in many forms throughout lifetimes. My most beautiful friend, thank you for being you – you are generous and kind and a joy to be around and I love you and cherish our friendship! Thanks also for all the words and for all of the suggestions throughout the journey of this book, they were invaluable.

Gill.

The puppy sitter extraordinaire. Thank you for all of who you are and all of the support and encouragement you have provided along the journey. You are an angel on my path and I thank you for your kindness and generosity of spirit. May your light continue to shine and be a beacon for others to follow.

Don and Tyler Tolman.

Words cannot express my deep gratitude for all of what you share. Your wisdom is profound. Your teachings are sublime. Your generosity of spirit – divine! Thank you for being trailblazers and for allowing passengers to board. You guys ROCK!

Joe Cross.

Aussie. Aussie. Aussie!!! Thank you Joe for all of what you are doing and have done to help people find their way to a better, healthier life through juice fasting. I love your humour and the way you go about keeping it real for people. You are an inspiration!

A whole bunch of people, far too many to name.

For all of those who inquired about juice fasting, told me their stories, asked about my book, got curious, urged me on, sent me blessings, read my manuscript and helped me make changes and for all of those who actually gave fasting a go (or simply indulged me why I spoke at length about it) – I thank you. You inspired and motivated me more than you will ever know. Thank you. Thank you. Thank you.

"If I have seen further, it is by standing upon the shoulders of giants"
~ Sir Isaac Newton (1643 – 1727)

Sir Isaac Newton is widely recognised as one of the most influential scientists of all time and as a key figure in the scientific revolution. He was an English physicist and mathematician who was most famous for his law of gravitation.

Author Biography

Julianne turned to natural healing when both her parents died after a long and horrific battle fighting cancer. Fuelled by her desire to live a long and healthy life and to not follow in their footsteps, Julianne found much evidence in support of regular fasting. As a self-proclaimed foodie, she challenged herself to have nothing but juice for seven days, and found that not only did she not die without food, she actually felt better and fasting gave her a great tool to rid the body of toxins and to repair and rejuvenate at a cellular level. The greatest influence on her work has been Don and Tyler Tolman who are renowned for helping people to understand the power of self-care and Joe Cross, another Aussie making huge strides with his movie's *Fat, Sick and Nearly Dead*. Julianne lives in Melbourne, Australia and this is her story.

Printed in the United States
By Bookmasters